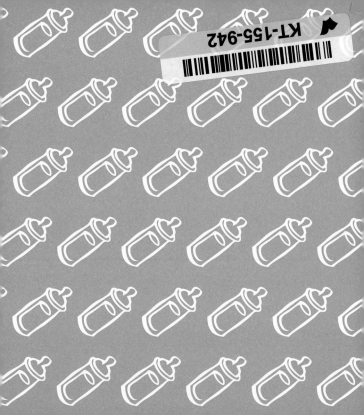

KT-155-942

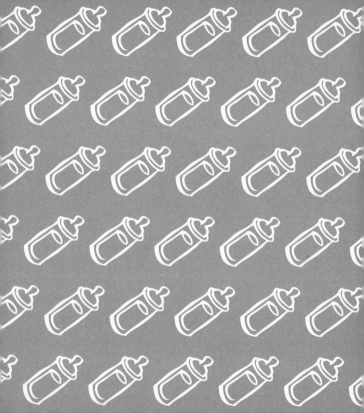

Baby Tips

for Dads

Simon Brett

Illustrations by
Alex Hallatt

summersdale

BABY TIPS FOR DADS

This edition published 2012

First published in 2004
Reprinted 2005, 2006 and 2007

Copyright © Simon Brett, 2004

Illustrations by Alex Hallatt

All rights reserved.

Summersdale Publishers Ltd
46 West Street
Chichester
West Sussex
PO19 1RP
UK

www.summersdale.com

Printed and bound in the Czech Republic

ISBN: 978-1-84953-283-9

Substantial discounts on bulk quantities of Summersdale books are available to corporations, professional associations and other organisations. For details contact Summersdale Publishers by telephone: +44 (0) 1243 771107, fax: +44 (0) 1243 786300 or email: nicky@summersdale.com.

To...

From...

Contents

Introduction

So there it is – your very own little baby. You are a dad. What a wonderful achievement! Granted, your partner may have made a greater contribution to the whole process, but your input was at least as important as hers – and a lot more fun.

So how are you going to cope with this new presence in your household? No amount of antenatal classes or concentrated reading of childcare manuals can prepare you for the reality of a baby. This little book, however, will give you some useful tips on how to face the challenges ahead.

How to Play the
Perfect Partner

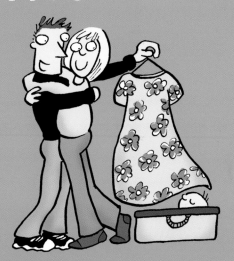

Things to say to your partner after she's had a baby:

'You've done enough by having the baby – I'll do everything else.' (It's a very tactful wheeze to say this. Doing it is a different matter entirely.)

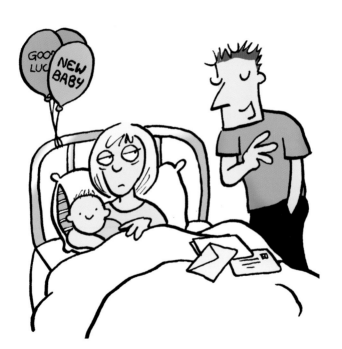

Things to say to your partner
after she's had a baby:

'I really think you look
thinner since you've had
the baby.'

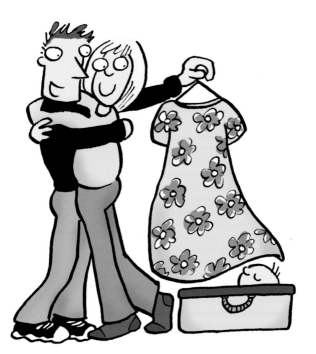

Things to say to your partner
after she's had a baby:

'I'll be happy to babysit
whenever you want to go
out for a girlie night with
your friends.'

Things to say to your partner
after she's had a baby:

'You need your sleep. I'll go
into the spare room next to
the nursery, and I'll get up
if the baby wakes in
the night.'

Things to say to your partner
after she's had a baby:

'Don't worry about me —
we'll get our sex-life back
on track when you feel like
it. No hurry.'

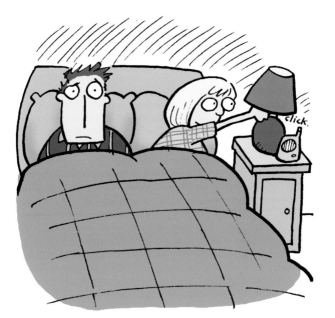

Things to say to your partner
after she's had a baby:

'We'll get an au pair.'

Things not to say to your partner after she's had a baby:

'Ooh look – a stretch-mark!'

Things not to say to your partner
after she's had a baby:

'Phwoar, look at
that woman over there –
her stomach's like an
ironing board.'

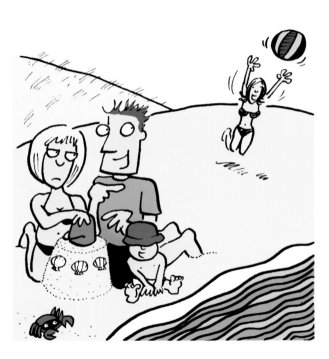

Things not to say to your partner
after she's had a baby:

'The baby's birth was
relatively easy.'

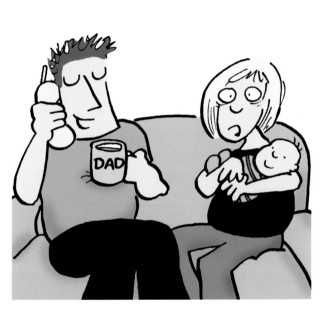

Things not to say to your partner
after she's had a baby:

'I don't think you've got
very much fatter.'

Things not to say to your partner
after she's had a baby:

'You always did have good
child-bearing hips.'

Things not to say to your partner
after she's had a baby:

'She's not with me.' (Said
when your partner starts
breast-feeding in public.)

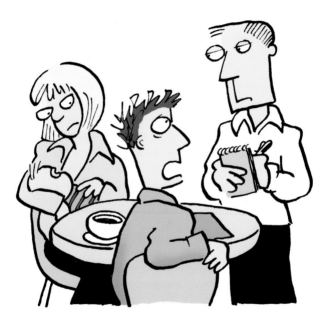

Things not to say to your partner
after she's had a baby:

'No one expects a woman's
breasts to be quite so firm
and pert after she's had
a baby.'

And don't say this one
at any time:

'You are getting to look
more and more like
your mother.'

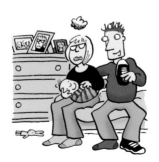

Signs your partner is spending too much time with the baby:

She pours your just-back-from-work Scotch into a sippy cup.

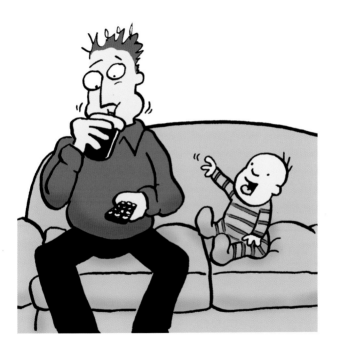

Signs your partner is spending too
much time with the baby:

She puts a bib on you
before serving your dinner.

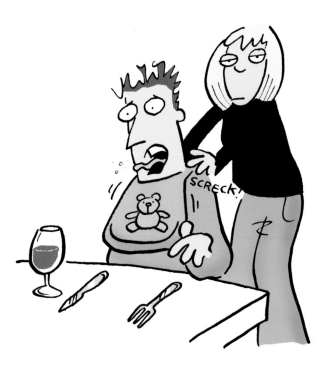

Signs your partner is spending too much time with the baby:

She cuts up the food of the person next to her at a dinner party.

Always agree:

When your partner says your baby is prettier/more intelligent/more advanced than anyone else's baby.

Always agree:

That your baby looks
exactly like whichever
relative happens to be
in the room at any
given moment.

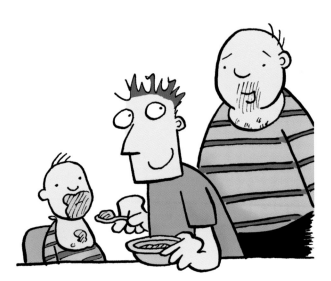

Always agree:

With your mother-in-law.
Well, at least try! Unless
of course you're in the
room when your partner
and mother-in-law are
discussing childcare and
want you to take sides. In
that case, go down the pub.

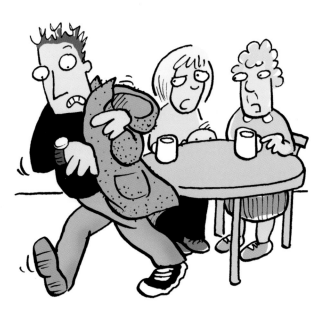

Always agree:

With your partner's views on childcare (so long as they don't involve you doing too much).

Daddy Dos and Don'ts

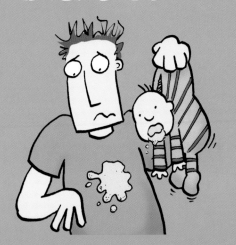

Under no circumstances be
heard to say any of
the following
(you'll regret it if you do):

'The baby's going to have to
fit into our routine.'

Under no circumstances be
heard to say any of the following
(you'll regret it if you do):

'I will never allow any baby
of mine to...' (Fill in the
blank. Whatever you say,
of course you will.)

Under no circumstances be
heard to say any of the following
(you'll regret it if you do):

'The baby's never
been carsick.'

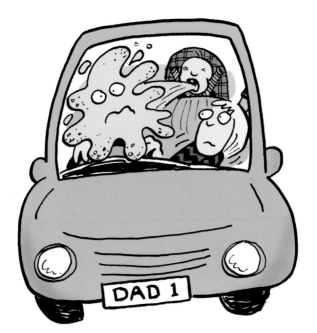

Under no circumstances be
heard to say any of the following
(you'll regret it if you do):

'We've been very lucky
with the baby sleeping
through the night.'

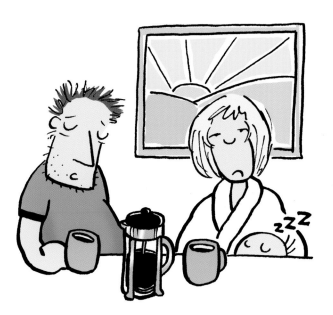

Under no circumstances be
heard to say any of the following
(you'll regret it if you do):

'We're certainly not going
to let having a baby affect
our sex life.'

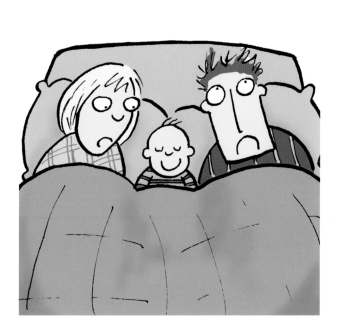

Under no circumstances be
heard to say any of the following
(you'll regret it if you do):

'I don't know why people
make such a big deal about
having a baby.'

Try to see things from your baby's point of view. Then you will understand that:

The sole purpose of your eyes is to have fingers poked into them.

Try to see things from your baby's point of view. Then you will understand that:

The sole purpose of your hair is to have baby food mashed into it.

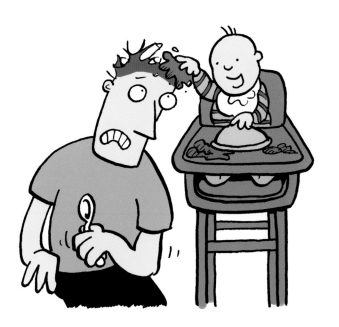

Try to see things from your baby's point of view. Then you will understand that:

The sole purpose of your clothes is to be puked over.

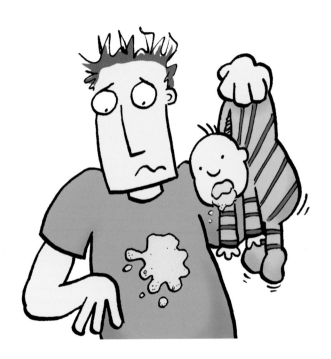

Your baby regards it as a solemn duty to stop you from doing any of the following:

Forgetting for a moment that you have a baby.

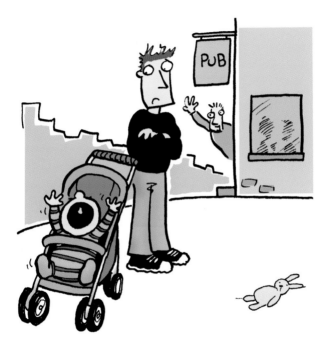

Your baby regards it as a solemn duty
to stop you from doing any of
the following:

Getting its clothes on.

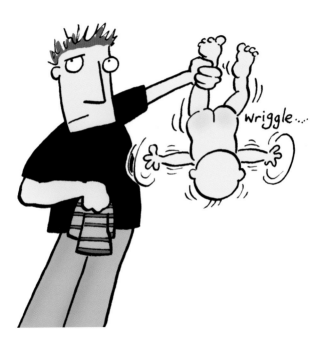

wriggle....

Your baby regards it as a solemn duty
to stop you from doing any of
the following:

Getting its nappy on.

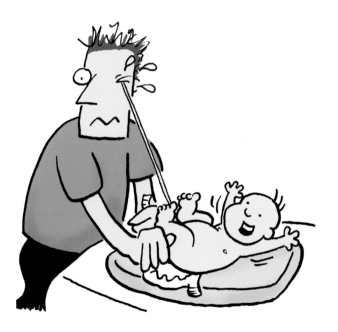

Your baby regards it as a solemn duty
to stop you from doing any of
the following:

Having a social life.

Your baby regards it as a solemn duty
to stop you from doing any of
the following:

Having a sex life.

Your baby regards it as a solemn duty
to stop you from doing any of
the following:

Sleeping.

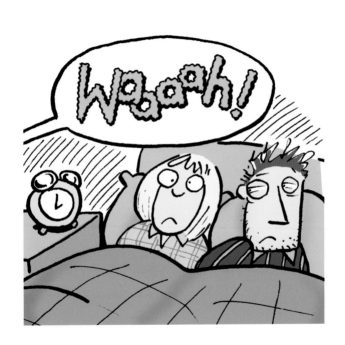

Baby Proverbs
for New Dads

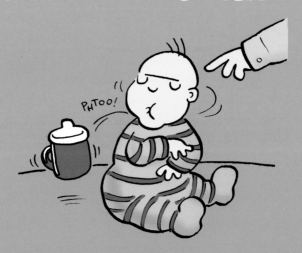

Baby proverbs for new dads:

What you lose on the swings you lose on the roundabouts – you have to keep on pushing on both of them.

Baby proverbs for new dads:

Cleanliness is next
to impossible.

Baby proverbs for new dads:

People who live in glass
houses with babies have
very smeary windows.

Baby proverbs for new dads:

A bad father blames
his tool.

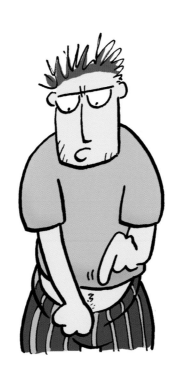

Baby proverbs for new dads:

The early baby catches the
worm... and then eats it.

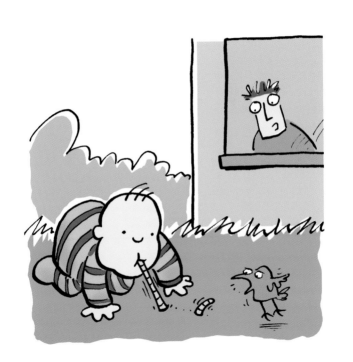

Baby proverbs for new dads:

One hour's sleep before midnight is all a parent's likely to get.

Baby proverbs for new dads:

Two's company, then you
have a baby.

Baby proverbs for new dads:

You can take a baby to the sippy cup, but you cannot make it drink.

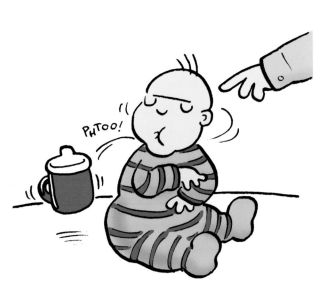

Baby proverbs for new dads:

It's an ill wind that needs
the most burping.

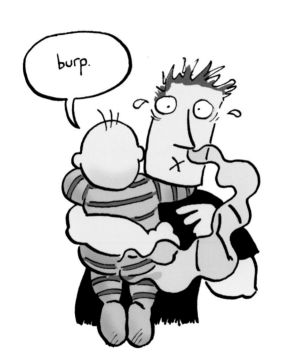

Baby proverbs for new dads:

Where there's a will,
there's frequently a rather
interesting choice of
baby's name.

Glossary of Useful Terms for New Dads

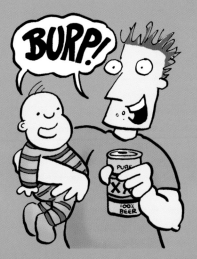

Glossary of useful terms for new dads:

ALLERGY: That which distinguishes the spots of middle-class children from those of lower-class children.

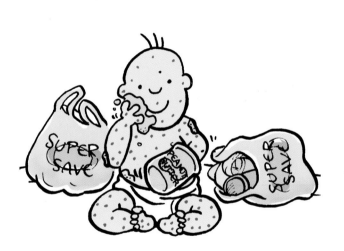

Glossary of useful terms
for new dads:

BURPING: An activity
passionately encouraged
in children until they are
weaned, and thereafter
equally passionately
discouraged.

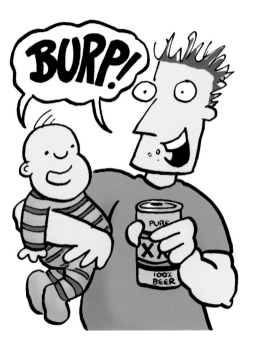

Glossary of useful terms
for new dads:

COITUS INTERRUPTUS: The
effect of children's
Sunday morning television
programmes finishing
earlier than the parents
thought.

Glossary of useful terms
for new dads:

CONSTIPATION: A no-go
situation. cf. DIARRHOEA: An
ongoing situation.

GLOSSARY OF USEFUL TERMS
FOR NEW DADS:

CONTRACTION: One of the
first signs of a baby's
arrival. The most notable
are contraction of space,
social life and spare cash.

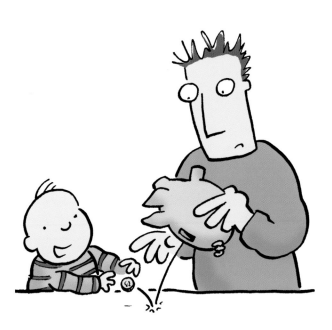

Glossary of useful terms
for new dads:

FAMILY PLANNING: Keeping
rival grandparents apart.

Glossary of useful terms
for new dads:

HEREDITY: The uncanny reappearance in children of all the good characteristics of one's own family and all the bad characteristics of one's in-laws.

Glossary of useful terms
for new dads:

IRON: A great help to the
well-being of the pregnant
and nursing mother. cf.
IRONING: No help at all to the
well-being of the pregnant
and nursing mother.

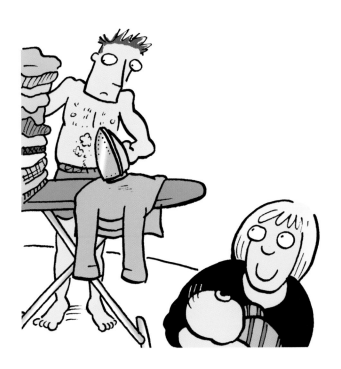

Glossary of useful terms
for new dads:

SUPPLEMENTARY FEEDING:
Baby's habit of coming into
parents' bed on Sunday
mornings and eating
the newspapers.

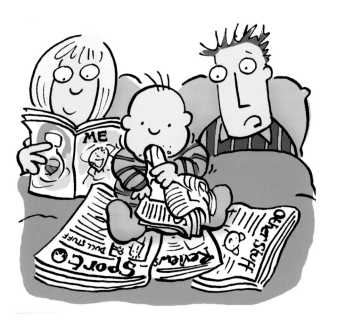

A final thought...

A baby is yours until it
leaves home, but your
partner's stretch marks
are forever.

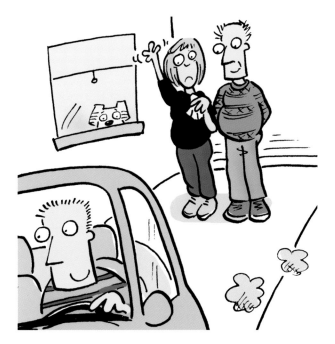

If you're interested in finding out more
about our humour books follow us
on Twitter: @SummersdaleLOL

www.summersdale.com

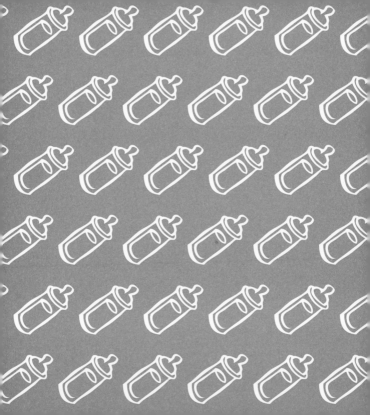

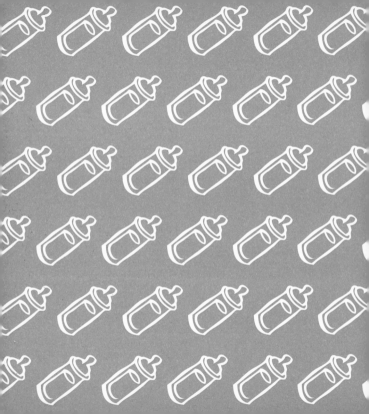